COMMON SENSE

MEDICARE FOR ALL
WHAT WILL IT MEAN FOR ME?

by
John Geyman, M.D.

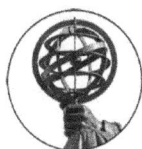

COPERNICUS
HEALTHCARE
Friday Harbor, WA

COMMON SENSE
MEDICARE FOR ALL
WHAT WILL IT MEAN FOR ME?

John Geyman, M.D.

Copernicus Healthcare
Friday Harbor, WA

First Edition

Booklet design, cover and illustrations by W. Bruce Conway
Author photo by Anne Sheridan

softcover: ISBN 978-1-938218-34-7
eBook ASIN:

Library of Congress Control Number is
Available Upon Request From the Publisher

Copernicus Healthcare
34 Oak Hill Drive
Friday Harbor, WA 98250

www.copernicus-healthcare.org

NOTE TO THE READER

In his famous pamphlet, *Common Sense*, written for the people of the Thirteen Colonies in 1775-1776, Thomas Paine made a strong case—based on *simple facts, plain arguments*, and *common sense*—to gain independence from England.

In this pamphlet, I also offer *simple facts, plain arguments*, and *common sense* about Medicare for All and how it can effectively address the failure of our present health care system to meet the needs of all Americans.

With many more COVID deaths than any other country in the world by population, the long-standing systemic problems of our health care system—decreased access to care based on ability to pay, not medical need; variable and often poor quality of care; and widespread disparities and inequities—have been exacerbated by the coronavirus.

The costs of health care and insurance continue to spiral upward in our corporatized, unaccountable non-system while the numbers of unemployed Americans without health insurance continue to grow unabated. Public health measures have been politicized and refused by many, delaying pandemic control, while many people forego care in ERs, clinics and hospitals due to fear of the virus or the costs of care.

Health care is now big business in the U. S., almost one-fifth of our GDP, a major player in the Fortune 500, and serving the needs of Wall Street and investors at the expense of patients, their families and taxpayers.

The incoming Biden administration faces daunting tasks. Three health reform alternatives will be debated: (1) building on the Affordable Care Act (ACA); (2) one or another variant of a public option; and (3) Medicare for All.

This pamphlet is intended to inform this debate, drawing on traditional American values, our experience over the years, and that of other advanced countries around the world. It is targeted to legislators in Congress, opinion leaders, grassroots activists, and all Americans seeking to better understand the alternatives and how they will affect their lives.

Table of Contents

COMMON SENSE
MEDICARE FOR ALL
WHAT WILL IT MEAN FOR ME?

I. Current Circumstances for Individuals, Families, and the Country

After almost one year into the COVID-19 pandemic, the U. S. population has seen devastating impacts that have changed everyday life for all of us, even to the point of economic survival for tens of millions of Americans. These markers show the extent of the new challenges for individuals and families at the start of 2021:

- More than 25 million COVID confirmed cases with more than 440,000 deaths.
- More than 100,000 residents and staff of long-term care facilities died of the coronavirus by Thanksgiving, about 40 percent of all COVID deaths in the country. [1]
- More than 40 million Americans filing for unemployment insurance for the first time, with many of those jobs not coming back.
- Increasing numbers of Americans without health insurance, well above the 30 million uninsured and 87 million underinsured before the pandemic.
- Growing numbers of people delaying or foregoing health care for a serious condition because of unaffordable costs, more than the record 25 percent before the pandemic. [2]

These additional markers indicate the severity of impacts on our country as a whole:

- The pandemic is still out of control, with record surges in COVID cases, hospitalizations and deaths spiking after the 2020 Thanksgiving and Christmas holidays.

- Basic public health measures, such as face masks and social distancing, have been politicized, thereby delaying pandemic control and increasing COVID deaths.
- Increasing numbers of Americans living in poverty, beyond the 43 million before the pandemic struck. [3]
- Proposed federal budget cuts for Medicare and Medicaid, Social Security, Planned Parenthood, and other essential programs. [4]
- Extreme income inequality with the richest 1% holding more of the nation's wealth than the bottom 90% of us. [5]
- Increasing inequities, with minorities more vulnerable in today's economic downturn, such as by having lower-wage jobs (if employed), higher unemployment rates, less able to work from home, and having higher death rates from COVID (eg., African-Americans with twice the mortality rate than whites). [6]
- Inadequate stimulus relief funds after prolonged inability of Congress and the Trump administration to enact relief. [7]
- Profiteering by corporate interests in the medical-industrial complex, including increasing costs of prescription drugs, exploitive prices for face masks and COVID test kits, and diversion of small business loans under the Paycheck Protection Program to Wall Street investors through dividends and stock buybacks. [8]
- Unprecedented polarization and distrust across society, likely based on ethnic segregation, economic inequality, corruption, and political polarization. [9]

These words by William Rivers Pitt, senior editor and leading columnist at *Truthout*, are spot on at this juncture:

> *Yes, the new year could be worse. Probably, it will be just as bad at least, unless our luck changes. Maybe, just maybe, it will be better, but only if we get out of our own way for once and let common sense and science drive the bus for a few blocks.* [10]

References:

1. COVID-19 has killed more than 100,000 residents and staff of long-term care facilities. *Kaiser Family Foundation*, November 25, 2020.
2. Saad, L. More Americans delaying medical treatment due to cost. *Gallup*, December 9, 2019.
3. Powers, N. Fear of a black planet: Under the Republican push for welfare cuts, racism boils. *Truthout*, January 21, 2018.
4. Proposed policy, payment, and quality provisions changes to the Medicare Physician Fee Schedule for Calendar Year 2021. CMS.gov. August 3, 2020.
5. Hightower, J. It's time for a (teeny) tax on wealth. *The Hightower Lowdown* 21 (8): 1-2, September 2019.
6. Morath, E, Omeokwe, A. Virus obliterates black job market. *Wall Street Journal*, June 10, 2020.
7. Lobosco, K, Luhby, T. Here's what's in the second stimulus package. *CNN Politics*, December 20, 2020.
8. Gregg, A. Firms paid dividends after getting PPP loans. *The Washington Post*, September 25, 2020: A 16.
9. Vallier, K. Why are Americans so distrustful of each other? *Wall Street Journal*, December 19-20, 2020.
10. Pitt, WR. In 2020, COVID put a mirror up to our society. *Truthout*, January 1, 2021.

II. Failure of the Private Health Insurance Industry

World War II was the main stimulus for the rapid development of employer-sponsored health insurance (ESI). It grew rapidly in a wartime economy that brought the country out of the Great Depression and into a severe labor shortage. By 1950, more than one-half of Americans were covered for the first time. [1]

An enormous profit-driven industry has since evolved, and today ESI is its dominant part involving some 150 million Americans. However, it has priced itself above what many individuals, families and employers can afford. Premiums and deductibles have increased rapidly over the last 10 years, much above workers' wages. [2] Figure 1 shows how our 5 largest private health insurers (Aetna, Anthem, Cigna, Humana and United Healthcare) are being kept afloat by federal support of privatized Medicare and Medicaid, in an increasing way, from 2010 to 2016. [3] Overpayments are widespread for both of these privatized plans, with duplicative payments common in more than 30 states. [4] Moreover, they provide worse quality of care than their not-for-profit counterparts. [5]

FIGURE 1

MEDICARE AND MEDICAID KEEP PRIVATE INSURERS AFLOAT

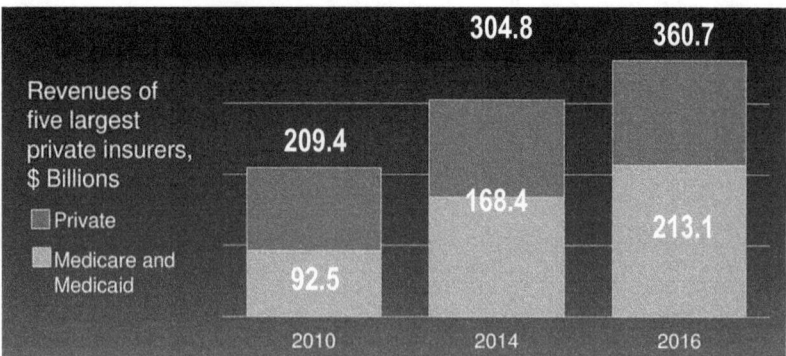

Source: *Health Affairs*; 36 (2):185, 2017

These are additional reasons that the industry no longer serves the public interest and should be retired:

- Even before the pandemic, employment was too volatile for reliable ESI, since people have held on average of 12 jobs on reaching age 50; in 2018, 66 million Americans left or lost their jobs, with many not regaining insurance in another job. [6]
- General Motors stopped paying health care premiums for 49,000 striking workers in 2019. [7]
- Small business, by far the most prevalent of businesses on Main Street, typically cannot afford to provide ESI to their employees, even in good times.
- Private health insurers restrict choice through narrowing of networks of physicians and hospitals. [8]
- The average time spent by physicians and their staffs each week to obtain prior authorization for tests or treatments is 14.6 hours, or about two work days. [9]
- The average denial rate for in-network claims across the industry is 18 percent. [10]
- Private health insurers continue to game the system at patients' expense through higher deductibles and copays, limited drug formularies, and deceptive marketing practices.
- Private health insurers exit unprofitable markets, often on short notice, leaving enrollees in the lurch.
- Greed is rampant in the industry; one of many examples is a proposed 2020 fine of $225 million by the Federal Communications Commission against Texas-based telemarketers for making about 1 billion illegally spoofed robocalls trying to sell short-term, limited duration health insurance plans. [11]
- The private health insurance industry has been bailed out for many years by the federal government, with continuing federal subsidies that average $685 billion a year. [12]

Wendell Potter, former Vice President of corporate communications at CIGNA and author of *Deadly Spin: An Insurance Company Insider Speaks Out on How Corporate PR is Killing Health Care and Deceiving Americans*, summarizes the case against ESI in this way:

> *America needs to get out of the business linking health insurance to job status. Even in better times, this arrangement was a bad idea from a health perspective. Most Americans whose families depend on their employers for coverage are just a layoff away from being uninsured. And now, when many businesses are shutting down and considering layoffs, it's a public health disaster.* [13]

References:

1.   Hacker, JS. *The Great Risk Shift: The Assault on American Jobs, Families, Health Care and Retirement and How You Can Fight Back.* New York. *Oxford University Press*, 2006, p. 145.
2.   Mathews, AW. Cost of employer health plans jumps. *Wall Street Journal*, September 29, 2019.
3.   Schoen, C, Collins, SR. The Big five health insurers' membership and revenue trends: Implications for public policy. *Health Affairs* 36 (2): December, 2017.
4.   National Health Expenditure Data—Historical. Centers for Medicare and Medicaid Services.
5.   Himmelstein, DU, Woolhandler, S, Hellander, I et al. Quality of care in investor-owned vs not-for-profit HMOs. *JAMA* 282: 159, 1999.
6.   Bruenig, M. People lose their employer-sponsored insurance constantly. *People's Advocacy Project*, April 4, 2019.

7. Johnson, J. Progressives say GM's decision to cut off employee health insurance yet another reason why we need Medicare for All. *Common Dreams*, September 18, 2019.

8. Rosenthal, E. *An American Sickness: How Healthcare Became Big Business and How You Can Take It Back.* New York. *Penguin Press*, 2017, pp, 235-236.

9. AMA Prior Authorization Physician Survey, December 2017.

10. Silvers, JB. This is the most realistic path to Medicare for All. *New York Times*, October 16, 2019.

11. FCC proposes record $225 million fine for massive spoofed robocall campaign selling health insurance. *Corporate Crime Reporter* 34 (24): June 15, 2020.

12. Ockerman, E. It costs $685 billion a year to subsidize U. S. health insurance. *Bloomberg News*, May 23, 2018.

13. Potter, W. Why the private health insurance industry faces an existential crisis. *The Progressive Populist*, November 1, 2019, p. 9.

III. What Will Medicare for All Mean for Me?

If I already have health insurance through my employer?
If I just lost my job?
If I am uninsured?
If I am underinsured?
If I am on Medicaid?
If I am in the Medicaid coverage gap?
If have pre-existing conditions?
If I own a small business?
If I already am on Medicare or have Medicare Advantage?
If I need long-term care?
If my income is below the federal poverty level?
If I have just gone through bankruptcy?

In all of these situations, the answer is good news!

When single-payer Medicare for All is enacted, everyone in the above circumstances will immediately be covered by a new system of national health insurance based on medical need, not ability to pay. These are components of that new coverage:

- Includes outpatient and inpatient services; laboratory and diagnostic services; dental, hearing and vision care; prescription drugs; reproductive health; maternity and newborn care; mental health services; and long-term care and supports. Coverage will extend to all 50 states, the District of Columbia, and U. S. territories.

- All U. S. residents will have full choice of physicians, other health professionals, hospital and other facilities. There will be no cost-sharing at the point of care, since everyone will have paid into the program all along.

- Employers of small businesses with less than 20 employees, representing 88 percent of all businesses on Main Street, will pay much less than they do now since their employees will already be covered with health insurance. [1]

- Administrative simplification with efficiencies and cost-containment through large-scale cost controls, including (a) negotiated fee schedules for physicians and other health professionals, who will remain in private practice; (b) global annual budgeting of hospitals and other facilities; and (c) bulk purchasing of drugs and medical devices.

- Cost savings that enable universal coverage through a not-for-profit public financing system.

- Sharing of risk for the costs of illness and accidents across our entire population of 330 million Americans. [2]

How much will I pay for Medicare for All?

As *individuals* at the point of care, you will find either no cost sharing or very minimal payments depending on the final legislation for Medicare for All. In either event, it will be much less than today's deductibles and copays.

As *small business owners*, you will pay much less than you do now, gain a healthier workforce, and be better able to survive the pandemic.

Then there is the question as to what happens with our taxes and spending for health care. One leading study by a team of economists at the University of Massachusetts Amherst's Political Economy Research Institute (PERI) compares the change in health care spending by income level with the existing system and Medicare for All (Figure 2). [3]

FIGURE 2

Percent Change in Health Care Spending Under Medicare for All by Income Level and Insurance Status, 2016

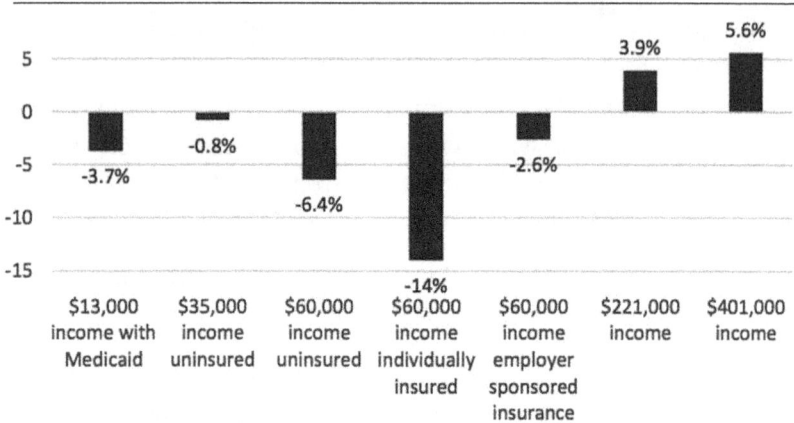

Sources: 2016 American Community Survey, the Consumer Expenditure Survey, and others.

If we were already individually insured with an annual income of $60,000, we would spend 14 percent less on health care than with the existing system, all without any pre-authorizations or denial of claims. Those with incomes above $221,000 would pay more (by 3.9 percent) while those above $401,000 would pay 5.6 percent more.

References:

1. Bivens, J. Medicare for All would boost workers' wages, expand workers' options, and likely create jobs. *Economic Policy Institute*, March 5, 2020.

2. Geyman, JP. *Common Sense: The Case For and Against Medicare for All: Leading Issue in the 2020 Elections*. Friday Harbor, WA. *Copernicus Healthcare*, 2019, pp. 3-4.

3. Pollin, R, Heintz, J, Arno, P et al. *In-depth analysis by team of UMass Amherst Economists shows viability of Medicare for All*. Amherst, MA, November 30, 2018.

IV. What will Medicare for All Mean for Our Country?

We have had a number of excellent national studies that have come to the same conclusion about Medicare for All—it will save us an immense amount of money while extending universal coverage to our entire population with much improved health outcomes. Cost estimates and savings vary somewhat depending on how progressive taxes are set up, but that conclusion holds fast.

Gerald Friedman, Professor of Economics at the University of Massachusetts Amherst, has studied the costs of Medicare for All over the last 10 years. He has found that we would have saved more than $1 trillion in 2019 had we had it in place that year. Figure 3 shows how these savings would have occurred, in billions, for three large areas of health care spending—provider administration (the billing process); insurance administration (interaction with private multi-payer insurers); and reduction to Medicare negotiated rates for payments to hospitals, drug companies, and medical equipment manufacturers (through bulk purchasing and negotiated prices). [1]

FIGURE 3

MEDICARE FOR ALL SAVINGS COMPARED TO CURRENT SYSTEM, 2019

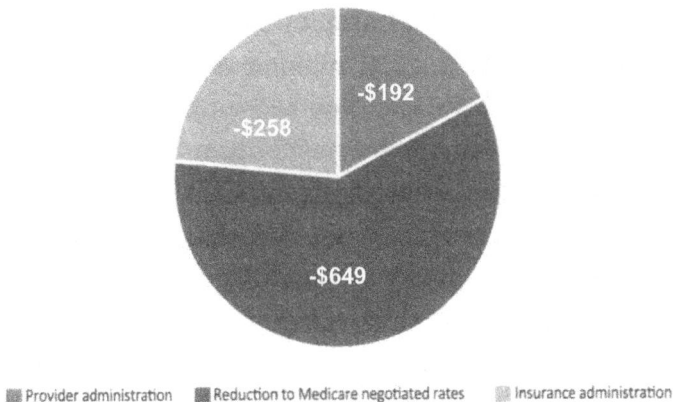

Provider administration   Reduction to Medicare negotiated rates   Insurance administration

Source: Friedman, E. *The Case for Medicare for All*. Medford, MA, *Polity Press*, 2020, p. 62.

The two major studies by economists at the University of Massachusetts Amherst (Friedman and PERI) used different assumptions for progressive taxes (Table 1) [2], but came to the same conclusion—Medicare for All can be readily paid for by savings plus moderate progressive taxes.

TABLE 1

RECOMMENDED PROGRESSIVE TAXES BY TWO STUDIES OF MEDICARE FOR ALL

FRIEDMAN STUDY	PERI STUDY
1. Tobin tax of 0.5% on stock trades and 0.01% per year to maturity on transactions in bond, swaps, and trades. 2. 6% surtax on household incomes over $225,000. 3. 6% tax on property income from capital gains, dividends, interest, or profits. 4. 6% payroll tax on top 60% with incomes over $53,000. 5. 3% payroll tax on bottom 40% with incomes under $53,000.	1. Business premiums set at 8 percent below what a business now spends on health care. 2. 3.75 percent sales tax on nonessential goods. 3. Recurring tax of 0.36 percent on all wealth over $1 million. 4. Taxing long-term capital gains as regular income.

Two other major national studies come to the same conclusion about Medicare for All. A recent Yale University study estimated that Medicare for All will prevent 68,000 deaths a year, together with saving more than $450 billion annually. [3]

Even more recently, the Congressional Budget Office (CBO) came out with another study that shows that Medicare for All will save us hundreds of billions annually. Its option that most closely approximates other studies, with low payment rates and low cost-sharing, is projected to save $650 billion in 2030; if long-term care and supports are added to benefits, savings would still be $300 billion in that year. [4]

Yes, high-income Americans will pay more in taxes when Medicare for All is implemented, but those increases are minimal compared to their tax rates from the 1920s up to 1970. (Figure 4) [5]

FIGURE 4

AVERAGE TAX RATES FOR THE TOP 0.1% VS. BOTTOM 90%, 1913-2020

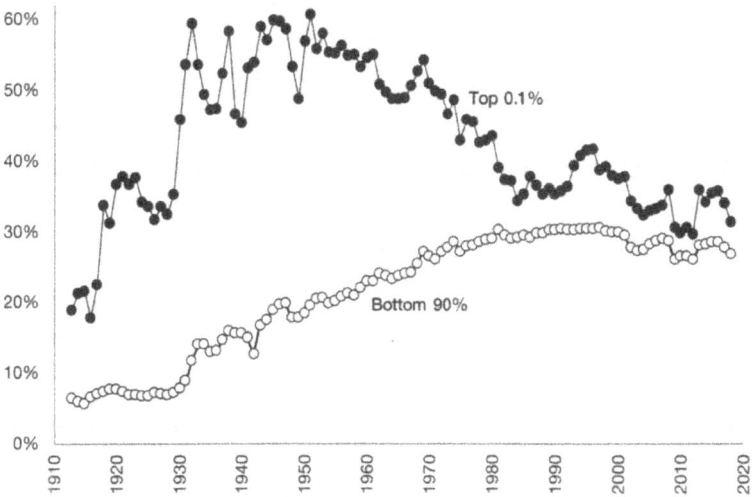

Source: Saez, E, Zucman, G. *The Triumph of Injustice: How the Rich Dodge Taxes and How to Make Them Pay*. New York. *W. W. Norton & Company*, 2019, p. 42.

Facing the future, there is already plenty of money in the system. It is not widely known that the government, through our taxes, already pays for *two-thirds* of U. S. health care spending.[6] Meaningful reform should be possible by redistributing money within a new system that reduces bureaucracy and waste and eliminates corruption. We should be able to achieve universal coverage and get a much better system for less money with Medicare for All.

These are some of the other advantages gained by Medicare for All at the national level as we continue to bring the COVID-19 pandemic under control:

- The 28-plus million Americans testing positive for CO-VID will receive necessary care.
- The labor market and economy will be helped by allowing employers to redirect money they have been spending on health care to their employees' wages. [7]
- Small business, which represents 88 percent of all businesses on Main Street, with less than 20 employees and less than $100,000 in annual revenue and are threatened with closure during this pandemic, will have their employees covered by health insurance. [8]
- The poverty level can be reduced by more than 20 percent by eliminating cost-sharing, self-payments and other out-of-pocket costs for health care. [9]

References:

1. Friedman, E. *The Case for Medicare for All*. Medford, MA. *Polity Press*, 2020, pp. 62-63.
2. Geyman, JP. *Common Sense: The Case for and Against Medicare for All. Leading Issue in the 2020 Elections*. Friday Harbor, WA. *Copernicus Healthcare,* 2019, p. 10.
3. Galvani, AP, Parpia, AS, Foster, EM et al. Improving the prognosis of health care in the USA. *Lancet* 395 (10223), February, 2020.
4. Bruenig, M. A new Congressional Budget Office study shows that Medicare for All would save hundreds of billions of dollars annually. *Jacobin Magazine*, December 19, 2020.
5. Saez, E, Zucman, G. *The Triumph of Injustice: How the Rich Dodge Taxes and How to Make Them Pay*. New York. *W. W. Norton & Company*, 2019, p. 42.

6. Himmelstein, DU, Woolhandler, S. The current and projected taxpayer shares of U. S. health care costs. *Amer J Public Health* on line, January 21, 2016.

7. Bivens, J. Fundamental health reform like 'Medicare for All' would help the labor market. *Economic Policy Institute*, March 5, 2020.

8. Matthews, C. Small business Administration touts $250 billion loan approvals, but there's little evidence small businesses are seeing cash. *Market Watch*, April 16, 2020.

9. Bruenig, M. Medicare for All would cut poverty by over 20 percent. *Peoples' Policy Project*, September 12, 2019.

V. Three Reform Alternatives and Why Medicare for All is the *Only* One that Will Work

The status quo is completely untenable in the aftermath of the Trump administration and in the midst of the most serious public health crisis since the 1918 influenza pandemic. We saw multiple efforts by Trump and the Republican-controlled Senate to dismantle the Affordable Care Act (ACA), including elimination of the individual mandate as part of the December 2017 GOP tax bill. That led to premium hikes by private insurers for their ACA plans and more people dropping their insurance. [1]

We now have a very corporatized and privatized non-system bent on raking in profits for Wall Street investors with little regard for the common good. Increasing privatization and profiteering by public programs have taken place, now including two thirds and three quarters of Medicare and Medicaid, respectively. Policies of the Trump administration allowed insurers to market short-term plans without the ACA's protections for pre-existing conditions and increase profits by counting their administrative and marketing costs as "direct patient care." They also permitted states to set work requirements for Medicaid beneficiaries (when most were already working!), impose lifetime caps on Medicaid benefits, and reduce or eliminate retroactive coverage of testing and treatment for COVID-19 and other medical care. [2] These policies have decimated what safety net we used to have, especially in lower-income urban settings and rural areas.

In the absence of a GOP health plan (despite several years of hearing that it was imminent!), we have just three major reform alternatives before us.

1. Build on the Affordable Care Act.

While centrists in the Biden administration favor this approach, including lowering the eligibility age for Medicare to 60, these are some of the many reasons that keeping the Affordable Care Act will not succeed:

- "It has failed to contain costs, and will continue to do so since a profiteering, inefficient private insurance industry is left in place.
- Insurance and health care will remain unaffordable and inaccessible for a large part of our population.
- COVID-19 care will not be fully covered.
- Continued inequities, with many Americans still delaying or foregoing essential care.
- Health insurance still pricey and volatile as employer-sponsored coverage is further stressed.
- Regulation of network size has been inadequate, as has gaming of the system by insurers.
- Many insurers abandon markets that are not sufficiently profitable, often with little advance notice.
- A continued Medicaid coverage gap exists in the states that refused to expand Medicaid." [3]

2. Variants of a Public Option

Several alternatives were put forward along the campaign trail in the recent election campaigns, including a public option alongside private plans on the ACA's exchanges, a Medicare Advantage for All plan, and lowering the eligibility age for Medicare.

In effect, each of these proposals would end up as Medicare for Some. Their advocates tout these approaches as more politically feasible, but none would adequately reform our system, for these reasons:

- Increased administrative complexity, costs, bureaucracy, and waste.
- Restricted access to care through private insurance networks.
- Non-comprehensive benefits.
- Continued high deductibles and other kinds of cost-sharing. [4]
- Continued high numbers of uninsured—still at least 15 to 20 million under Biden's plan.
- Would sacrifice about $350 billion a year of Medicare for All's savings as well as another $220 billion a year in private insurers overhead expenses. [5]

We already know from the last 10 years' experience that a public option won't work. A number of private non-profit CO-OPs were established under the ACA with the hope that they could compete, reduce cost, and increase the value of health insurance. They generated opposition from the insurance industry, most disappeared, and the few that remain cover just 1 percent of the 11 million ACA enrollees who got coverage through the exchanges. [6]

3. Medicare for All

This is the only way we can get out of this dysfunctional fix we are in with U. S. health care. Our financing system has failed over many years. We have seen earlier how Medicare for All will directly address serious system problems of access and financial barriers to care, unacceptable quality, persistent disparities and inequities, bureaucracy and waste. All of these ongoing problems have been exacerbated by the COVID-19 pandemic. Had we had a single-payer system of universal coverage at its outset, together with a well-funded public health infrastructure, we could have controlled the pandemic much earlier with far fewer lives lost and less disruption of our economy.

The fatal flaw against the first two alternatives is that they leave in place an obsolete private health insurance industry, with its dependence on a failing system of employer-sponsored coverage. Dr. Atul Gawande, surgeon, public health researcher, and author of *Being Mortal: Medicine and What Matters in the End,* brings us this important insight:

> *The central error of our system has been attaching our health care to where we work. A company-sponsored insurance plan for a family adds an average of fifteen thousand dollars to the annual cost of employing a worker—effectively levying a fifty-per-cent tax on a fifteen-dollar-an-hour position. We're all but paying employers to outsource or automate people's jobs. The result is to make both work and health care less secure and more fragmented—and to deepen our inequalities.[7]*

With Medicare for All, transition can be achieved with less disruption than occurs every day in our present fragmented, overly bureaucratic non-system. Administration will be greatly simplified at a much lower cost, perhaps as low as 1.5 percent by the CBO's analysis, compared to privatized Medicare Advantage's 13.7 percent administrative overhead. [8]

Disinformation about Medicare for All

Concerted opposition to Medicare for All from corporate stakeholders across the medical-industrial complex should not be underestimated. With their deep pockets and lobbyists (as many as five for every member of Congress) they seek to spread disinformation and build opposition to it based on these kinds of false assertions:

1. NHI will be a government takeover and bring socialism.

Under NHI, physicians and other health professionals would not be employed by the government but remain in private practice. Private hospitals and other facilities would retain their private ownership and receive global, year-to-year operating budgets. [9, 10] Medicare for All would join other taxpayer supported institutions in the public interest, such as fire and police departments, public schools, and our national parks.

2. Physicians won't like it.

On the contrary, they and other health professionals are beleaguered by the growing burden of contending with changing policies of insurers, such as restricted networks, changing drug formularies, pre-authorizations, and other requirements related to reimbursement. Now that two-thirds of physicians are employed by others, mostly hospital systems, and under the gun to bring higher revenues to their employers, growing numbers are retiring early. [11] A majority of U. S. physicians support Medicare for All, as does the 159,000-member American College of Physicians, the second largest physician organization in the country. [12]

3. The public doesn't want it.

National polls continue to find that more than two-thirds of the public support Medicare for All, including more than 80 percent of Democrats and even 52 percent of Republicans. A 2019 report from Gallup News documented that 70 percent of Americans have, over more than 20 years, described the U. S. health care system as being in a state of crisis over its decreased access, uncontrolled prices, and unpredictable quality of care. [13]

4. It will be too disruptive.

This scare tactic by opponents of Medicare for All and defenders of the status quo disregard how volatile private health insurance is, how frequently people lose their jobs and insurance, and how disruptive these frequent changes are for everyday Americans. On the flip side, all Americans will have continuous health insurance under Medicare for All, with much less disruption in their lives.

Table 2 compares the three major alternatives for health care reform based on evidence. [14]

TABLE 2

COMPARISON OF THREE REFORM ALTERNATIVES BASED ON EVIDENCE

	ACA	PUBLIC OPTION	MEDICARE for ALL
Access	Restricted	Restricted	Unrestricted
Choice	Restricted	Restricted	Unrestricted
Cost containment	Never	Never	Yes
Quality of care	Unacceptable	Unacceptable	Improved
Bureaucracy	Increased	Increased	Much reduced
Universal coverage	Never	Never	Yes, immediately
Accountability	No	No	Yes
Sustainability	No	No	Yes

The biggest question concerning moving forward with real health care reform is political will. Dr. Peter Arno and Dr. Phillip Caper, physicians with long experience with health policy and previous failed reform attempts, offer us this penetrating observation:

The real struggle for a universal single payer system in the U. S. is not technical or economic but almost entirely political. Retaining anything resembling the status quo is the least disruptive, and therefore politically easier route. Unfortunately, it is also the least effective route to attack the underlying pathology of the American health care system— corporatism run amok. Adopting the easiest route will do little more than kick the can down the road and will require repeatedly revisiting the deficiencies in our health care system until we get it right. [15]

The stakes couldn't be higher as we try to get beyond the COVID-19 pandemic, rebuild our economy, and deal with the polarized politics of our time. The Biden administration has a unique opportunity to get it right on health care, almost 18 percent of our GDP. Do we dither and let the power and money of the medical-industrial complex win once again, or do we take this opportunity to build a 'new normal' that meets the needs of our country for equal opportunity and social justice?

After so many years of failed incremental attempts at health care reform, we now have the opportunity to take the rampant corporate profits out of our system and adopt Medicare for All, which addresses the common good. Medicare for All can be the social glue to bring us together. The survival of millions of Americans hangs in the balance, as does our democracy.

References:

1. Cunningham, PW. The Health 202: Your health policy appointment. *The Washington Post,* December 21, 2017.

2. Shafer, P, Huberfeld, N, Golberstein, E. Medicaid retroactive eligibility waivers will leave thousands responsible for coronavirus treatment costs. *Health Affairs Blog,* May 8, 2020.

3. Geyman, JP. *America's Mighty Medical-Industrial Complex: Negative Impacts and Positive Solutions.* Friday Harbor, WA. *Copernicus Healthcare,* 2021.

4. Himmelstein, DU, Woolhandler, S. The 'public option' on health care is a poison pill. *The Nation*, October 21, 2019.

5. Ibid # 4.

6. Galewitz, P. Kaiser Health News. Only three of 26 Obama-era non-profit health insurance co-ops will soon remain. *Fortune*, September 6, 2020.

7. Gawande, A. A Nation's Health Care: Rescuing the System. *The New Yorker,* October 5, 2020: pp. 12-13.

8. Bruenig, M. A new Congressional Budget Office study shows that Medicare for All would save hundreds of billions of dollars annually. *Jacobin Magazine*, December 19, 2020.

9. Potter, W. I used to be a propagandist for insurance companies. Learn the four truths the insurance industry doesn't want Americans to see. *Tarbell*, April 30, 2019.

10. Geyman, JP. Fact check on claims by opponents of Medicare for All. *Physicians for a National Health Program*, November 30, 2019.

11. Jones, VA. The reasons why so many physicians are retiring early. *MEDPAGE TODAY'S* Kevin MD.com, March 6, 2019.

12. Queally, J. In historic shift, second largest physicians group in U. S. has new prescription: It's Medicare for All. *Common Dreams*, January 20, 2020.

13. Gallup News, as referenced by Conley, J. New analysis shows why Democrats are wrong to fear bold embrace of Medicare for All. *Common Dreams*, January 14, 2019.

14. Geyman, JP. Common Sense: *Medicare for All: Foundation of a 'New Normal' in U. S. Health Care.* Friday Harbor, WA. *Copernicus Healthcare*, 2020, p. 23.

15. Arno, P, Caper, P. Medicare for All: The social transformation of U. S. health care. *Health Affairs*, March 25, 2020.

VI. Useful Resources

Websites
1. Physicians for a National Health Program (PNHP): www.pnhp.org
2. Quote of the Day. don@mccanne.org
3. HealthCare-NOW. www.healthcare-now.org
4. www. johngeymanmd.org

Reports
1. Overall Health System Performance in Eleven Countries. Periodic reports from *The Commonwealth Fund*, New York City, NY
2. Public Citizen. *The Case for Medicare for All*, Washington, D.C., February 4, 2019.
3. Bruenig, M. A new Congressional Budget Office study shows that Medicare for All would save hundreds of billions of dollars annually, *Jacobin Magazine*, December 19, 2020.

Books
1. Rosenthal, E. *An American Sickness: How Healthcare Became Big Business and How You Can Take It Back*. New York. *Penguin Press,* 2017.
2. Saez, E, Zucman, G. *The Triumph of Injustice: How the Rich Dodge Taxes and How to Make Them Pay*. New York. *W. W. Norton & Company, Inc*, 2019.
3. Friedman, G. *The Case for Medicare for All*. Medford, MA. *Polity Press*, 2020.
4. Geyman, JP. *America's Mighty Medical-Industrial Complex: Negative Impacts and Positive Solutions*. Friday Harbor, WA. *Copernicus Healthcare*, 2021.

Articles
1. Light, DW. A conservative call for universal access to health care. *Penn Bioeth J*, 9 (4): 4-6, 2002.
2. Arno, P, Caper, P. Medicare for All: The social transformation of U. S. health care. *Health Affairs*, March 25, 2020.
3. Archer, D, Potter, W. To defeat coronavirus, we need to expand Medicare. *Common Dreams*, June 8, 2020.
4. Himmelstein, DU, Woolhandler, S. The 'public option' on health care is a poison pill. *The Nation*, October 21, 2019.
5. Geyman, JP. What is the 'public option?' Can it compete with private health insurers? *CounterPunch*, January 8, 2021.
6. Gawande, A. A Nation's Health Care: Rescuing the System. *The New Yorker*, October 5, 2020: pp. 12-13.

ABOUT THE AUTHOR

John Geyman, M.D. is professor emeritus of family medicine at the University of Washington School of Medicine in Seattle, where he served as Chairman of the Department of Family Medicine from 1976 to 1990. As a family physician with over 21 years in academic medicine, he also practiced in rural communities for 13 years. He was the founding editor of *The Journal of Family Practice* (1973 to 1990) and the editor of *The Journal of the American Board of Family Medicine* from 1990 to 2003. Since 1990 he has been involved with research and writing on health policy and health care reform. He served as president of Physicians for a National Health Program from 2005 to 2007, and is a member of the National Academy of Medicine.

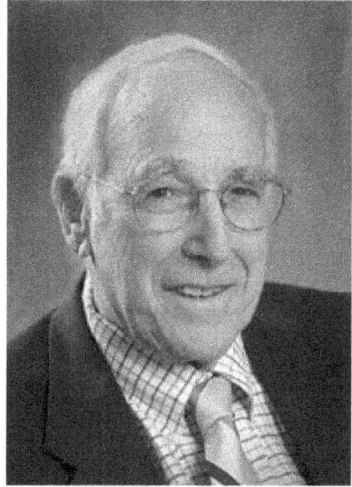

His books include:

Profiteering, Corruption and Fraud in U.S. Health Care (2020)

Common Sense: Medicare for All: Foundation of a 'New Normal' in U. S. Health Care (Pamphlet, 2020)

Long Term Care in America: The Crisis All of Us Will Face in Our Lifetimes, (2019)

Common Sense: The Case For and Against Medicare For All (Pamphlet, 2019)

Struggling and Dying Under TrumpCare: How We Can Fix this Fiasco (2019)

Trumpcare: Lies, Broken Promises, How it is Failing, and What Can Be Done (2018)

Common Sense: U. S. Health Care at a Crossroads in the 2018 Congress
(Pamphlet, 2018)

Common Sense about Health Care Reform in America
(Pamphlet, 2017)

Crisis in U.S Health Care: Corporate Power vs. the Common Good (2017)

*The Human Face of ObamaCare: Promises vs. Reality and What
Comes* Next (2016)

*How ObamaCare is Unsustainable: Why We Need a Single-Payer Solution
for All Americans* (2015)

*Souls on a Walk: An Enduring Love Story Unbroken by
Alzheimer's* (2012)

*Health Care Wars: How Market Ideology and Corporate Power Are Killing
Americans* (2012)

*Breaking Point: How the Primary Care Crisis Endangers the Lives of
Americans.* (2011)

*Hijacked: The Road to Single-Payer in the Aftermath of Stolen Health Care
Reform* (2010)

The Cancer Generation: Baby Boomers Facing a Perfect Storm (2009)

*Do Not Resuscitate: Why the Health Insurance Industry is Dying, and How
We Must Replace It* (2008)

The Corrosion of Medicine: Can the Profession Reclaim Its Moral Legacy?
(2008)

Shredding the Social Contract: The Privatization of Medicare (2006)

Falling Through the Safety Net: Americans Without Health Insurance (2005)

*The Corporate Transformation of Health Care: Can the Public Interest Still
Be Served?* (2004)

Health Care in America: Can Our Ailing System Be Healed? (2002)

Family Practice: Foundation of Changing Health Care (1985)

The Modern Family Doctor and Changing Medical Practice (1971)

Copies of this pamphlet can be ordered from Amazon.com for $5.95, or as a Kindle eBook version at $2.99.

For more background and analysis, copies of my new 2021 book, *America's Mighty Medical-Industrial Complex: Negative Impacts and Positive Solutions,* can also be ordered from Amazon.com ($18.95) or as a Kindle eBook ($5.99).